# REST

# MANIFESTO

## SAVASANA

## TO CHANGE THE WORLD

## Beth Bayley

But hey, thank you for buying it! A portion of the proceeds will go to charity to fight racism and support equality in the yoga community and beyond. More info will be on bethbayley.yoga

The Rest Manifesto: Savasana to Change the World / Beth Bayley.
—1st ed.
ISBN 978-1-953449-05-4

# CONTENTS

*For my darling BH*

# Introduction

## *Space for peace*

Savasana, the Sanskrit word for corpse pose, is the final resting pose of most hatha yoga classes. The sequence of moving through poses and then lying down at the end is familiar to most of us. This book is about spending more time in the lying-down part – why it matters, and what can happen when we do. This book is an invitation to a daily restorative savasana – a simple practice with profound effects.

A daily restorative savasana:

- Can help you integrate your body and your mind, allowing you to be more comfortable in your own skin.

- Can give you perspective on the issues in your daily life, and help you enjoy that daily life more.

- Can help you to become a better person – really! – and prepare you to take on the tasks of being a global citizen.

- Can lead to a little bit of samadhi, or bliss.

Whether you have been to a thousand yoga classes or none, whether you are a type A overachiever or a hermit in the woods, we all get stressed out and we all carry that stress within our bodies. We all think that getting more sleep will solve it, but sleep, if punctuated by bad dreams and a clenched jaw, isn't always restful. And even the best sleepers may have restless waking lives.

Yet you have the ability to breathe peace, or space for potential peace, inside your body, whenever you choose.

*Setting aside time every day to consciously relax will change your life.*

Does this sound too good to be true? It gets even more so:

Restorative savasana is appropriate and accessible for all bodies. And you don't need anything to do it. Well, maybe a timer. Maybe a mat and some pillows (but these are optional).

When practicing restorative yoga, you don't add things in – rather, you take them off. You remove your uncomfortable clothes, set aside your distracting tech.

You let your worries fall into the floor...and eventually your past, and your identity, too. All the stories you don't need slip away from you, so you can better understand the ones you do.

# My story

## *Design flaws*

**S**avasana has always come easily to me – probably too easily. My preschool teacher asked my parents[i] if I was getting enough sleep at home, because I liked to lie down during story time instead of sitting up with the other children.

"No, she's just like that," they said. "A little bit lazy."

And I continued being lazy (conserving my energy!), avoiding all exercise if I could help it, until I found yoga, taking my first hot power vinyasa class in 2000.[ii] For 20 years I practiced – and eventually taught – a very fitness-y and athletic style of yoga, as well as other movement classes. This was a perfect counterpoint for my innately slothful nature. I enjoyed it, and benefited from the movement, and obediently lay down for the last five minutes. Teachers would often say that savasana might be the hardest part for some of us, but also the most important. *It's not hard*, I thought. *But is it really important?*

Strenuous asana gave me the gifts of strength, discipline, and concentration. But in my own practice, I was always trying to "correct" something: my genetically crooked leg, my big thighs, my wobbly bakasana, my laziness. It wasn't until I found restorative yoga, and the meditative states that it allowed me to access, that I began to understand:

My crooked leg isn't a problem: it's a *gift*, from my mother, and her mother before her. My body is *supposed* to be this way: it was naturally selected for so many generations to be like this. *All the flaws are part of the design.*

AND THIS IS TRUE FOR EVERYONE. The flaws are part of the design – your task in this lifetime is to adapt to how you were built, adapt to your genes and your circumstances, and to use that adaptation to *do the things only you can do*. To fulfill your dharma, if you want to think of it that way.[iii]

Savasana was never hard for me. What was hard was self-acceptance. And this practice changed everything. Self-acceptance is the only way we can "get anywhere."[iv] The only way we can grow.

My hope is that this tiny book makes a daily restorative savasana a simple and accessible practice for everyone. I have outlined my own yoga philosophy, given a few variations of shapes to rest in, and offered some ideas for unknotting your tangled mind. Please take only what's useful for you.

# Don't resist/resist

## *Gathering strength through softening*

There are two kinds of resistance at play in our resting bodies.

When we spend time in savasana, softening our bodies and minds, we are like a river flowing, unresisting, over all the rocks and obstacles in our path, smoothing them out with time. Not resisting the way that things truly are can lead to great peace and a profound life-changing acceptance.

"Give me the strength to accept what I cannot change..." as the prayer goes. Not strength like a clenching fist or gritted teeth. Strength like the rushing river, the enduring mountain, and the wide open sea.

There's another kind of resistance: political resistance. It matters *so much*. And lying down is a political act.

- Every time we lie down and remember we are already okay, we are resisting a capitalist system that *needs us to believe we will never be good enough* in order for it to operate.

- Every time we lie down and remember we are already perfect, we are resisting the racist systems that *need us to hate ourselves and others* in order to operate.

- Every time we lie down and remember that the still small voice inside us, underneath the mean yammering one, is *who we truly are*, we are less likely to seek sustenance from the approval of friends and strangers, in life and online.

*The more we lie down, the more we will remember to love ourselves and each other.*

Lying down is NOT a substitute for activism, but a marvelous and necessary complement. We must lie down and rest so we can stand up and fight!

# The practice

## *Doing nothing*

**E**very day, for at least 20 minutes, lie down and do nothing.

*Nothing.*

You can do this in the morning to set the tone for your day, after work to separate public and domestic life, or in the evening to wind down before bed (though not if it means you'll just fall asleep in the pose – we are trying to stay awake).

You can do this after other yoga asanas, after other exercise, or simply whenever you feel like it.

It's easier for most bodies to come to stillness after moving the spine – plus it's great to do this every day, to keep your back healthy – so one option is to take a few moments to move the spine in all directions. A seated forward fold, a small arch back to open the chest, rotations, side bends, and twists, for a few breaths in each position, can be a part of the ritual of settling in.

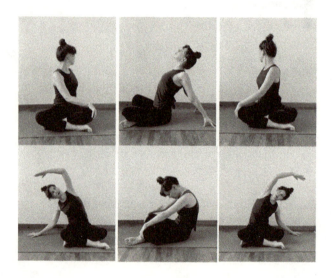

Find a space where you will not be disturbed, so that you can sustain the shape until you are ready to come out.

Light a candle, if that's your thing.

Set a timer, so you don't have to think about it.

Ensure that you will not be distracted by anything electronic.

Or by other people, as much as it is in your control.

Prop up your knees so they are softly bent, your head so it doesn't feel like it's tipping back, and your shoulders so they feel supported.

Surround yourself with more pillows and blankets, if you like, so you feel safe and cocooned.

Choose a shape that best suits you today...

Minimalist (head support only, knees falling together):

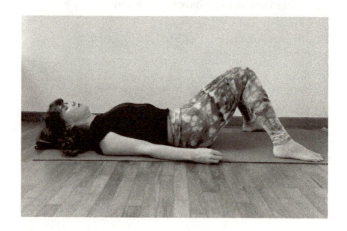

Some support (head and shoulders supported, bolster under bent knees) (this is my personal favorite option):

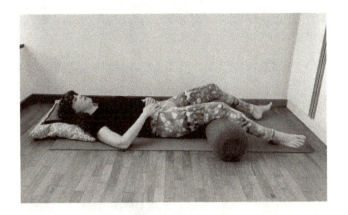

Maximalist (a.k.a. first class pose or massage chair pose, with a supported head and spine, covered eyes, bent knees, and elevated ankles):

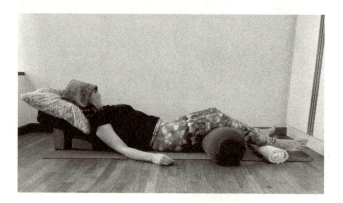

Assisted by the wall or furniture (a.k.a. viparita karani, minus any major stretch or strain):

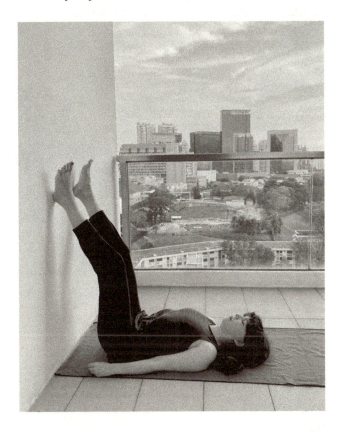

Or whatever (and wherever) else you can think of:

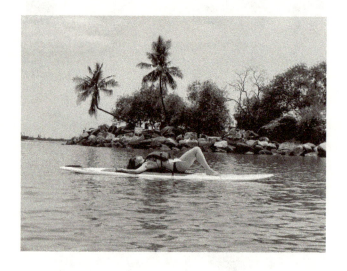

Take your time! If you aren't comfortable, you'll be like the princess and the pea, and it'll make you crazy. Adjust until you get there, until you feel safe in the space you have chosen, and held comfortably by the props around you.

Cover your eyes if you'd like. Perhaps rest your hands on your body to feel your breath.

And then let your breath be free, spacious, deep, and unhurried, completely unrestricted by clothes or position.

Then you are there. With nothing to fix. Nothing to do but melt like ice cream into the floor. Or you can be an ice cube, or butter, or anything else melty and pleasant.

Holding the world up is exhausting.

And defeating.

And unnecessary.

Let the world hold you.

# Your body: some science

## *Shifting over*

**W**hy 20 minutes? It's a reasonable container to set aside and fill with rest, as it's less than two percent of your entire day. It also takes about 20 minutes to shift all the way from fight or flight to rest and digest.

The Relaxation Response is the feeling that arises as the parasympathetic nervous system is engaged. [v] The PSNS assists with blood flow, long-term health, immunity, digestion, and reproduction. Its counterpart, where we spend a lot of unnecessary time, is the sympathetic nervous system, a.k.a. the SNS, a.k.a. the fight-flight-freeze response.

We need the SNS for our survival, as well as for many of the tasks of everyday life. But when we spend too long with the SNS activated, it's hard to be optimistic. Hard to see the big picture. Hard to connect with others. As we relax our tense muscles, our bodies' blood and resources are shared with all of our systems, not just the ones we need to respond to danger.

***

As you ease into the pose, keep in mind that you aren't trying for perfect stillness, or some kind of frozen holding in place. This is a release, so let yourself move and fidget until you get to comfort. Scan from your toes to your scalp, scalp to toes, and progressively relax your muscles (possibly choosing to flex them, one body part a time), if you still have a lot of restless energy.

Remember that this pose is not a stretch, but rather an intentional softening. A "conscious relaxation," as my teacher Adeline Tien says. As you begin to melt into the floor on your exhales, check in with your own energy.

Are you doing extra work in your body? Maybe pressing down into the props, or setting your jaw in a habitual tightness? (Do you always do extra work, in the rest of your life?). *See if you can let it go, just a little bit.* All you have to do is lie there, and the world will keep spinning just fine. This is the time for no efforting, no striving, no straining, no grasping. Just being as you are.

Which is unusual, right? To lie down without a goal. There are more physically challenging asanas, or all kinds of other things you may think you should do[vi] – but listen: being able to touch your toes won't get you into heaven. Or Harvard.

It's more interesting to think about *why* you want to do those other challenging things. How much is ego involved? What do you hope to accomplish, and when you accomplish it, what do you think will happen? Are you after some kind of perfection? Because you are already perfect! There is no need to grasp or strive.

You only need to lie down, soften your tension, feel your feelings, and when you stand up again, you'll be, subtly, changed.

More and more, every time.

# Your mind: some psychology

## *Inside/outside*

Research has found that thoughts, and the emotions attached to them, rise and fall away in 90-second wavelengths.[vii] If we choose to follow them, they last longer (ask any insomniac), but if we just watch them without engaging, they fall away in less than two minutes.

Thinking is natural – it's what the mind does. We are not trying for aggressive emptiness here. And there is no doing it "right" or "wrong." Your job is only to shift your attention from thinking to feeling. Then to feel your feelings and let them move through you.

Emotions can get stuck in our bodies. We all carry around icebergs of old thoughts and feelings and experiences and stories – but energy can't move through stuck or frozen tissue.[viii]

You must feel your feelings, the full range of whatever comes up, in order to move them through you. To breathe them out. This is how we build emotional resilience and strength – not by avoiding, or stuffing them down, but experiencing them.

So this melting-into-the-floor savasana is also a form of meditation, one in which you maintain a gentle curiosity for your thoughts. How is the energy inside your brain? Are you prone to rehashing past or rehearsing future conversations? Folding the laundry that's still in the dryer?

We all have collections of memories and experiences rattling around in the shoeboxes of our mind, or lodged firmly underneath the couch cushions of our subconscious. Lie still long enough and your mind will travel, sit on that couch, open those shoeboxes. Your mind will go to the past or the future (neither of which are really *real* right now) and all you have to do is notice where it goes. Does your mind travel to the same places all the time? Why is that?

Then – and this is important – notice what happens with your physical body when your mind goes somewhere. Perhaps your eyebrows furrow, your jaw tenses...and that's okay. Keep coming back to the body and softening the tension as you exhale, with patient and loving awareness.

This is not always easy. Sometimes it can be terrible.

But I promise it's always worth it.

Buddhist meditation teacher and psychologist Tara Brach says it best:

"In accepting the waves of thought and feeling that arise and pass away, we realize our deepest nature, our original nature, as a boundless sea of wakefulness and love."[ix]

# Bliss and the Yoga Sutras

## *Deeper inward*

Asana, or the physical poses of yoga, is just one of the 8 facets of the yogic way as described by the sage Sri Patanjali in the Yoga Sutras, probably around 100-200AD. Like many old and sacred texts, the Sutras are worthy of deep study and subject to interpretation – and what follows is my own opinion.

The Sutras are often described as a path, or a road map:[x] a guide for living a whole and meaningful life, as my teacher Sophie Sanders reminds us.

The Sutras' first four facets are the yamas (which are about personal integrity and ethics), the niyamas (about self-restraint and spiritual observances), asana (the poses), and pranayama (the breath). These four have to do with how we relate to the outer world, especially regarding our behavior and actions towards others. They also concern how we relate to ourselves, and how we choose to move and breathe within our bodies. The disciplined choices we make.[xi]

Sometimes while practicing savasana, we get lucky enough to spend time with the next four facets of yoga. These four concern the senses, the mind, and consciousness. These are special states – but they aren't reserved for special holy people. They are available to all of us. If you are a human with a heart and a soul, these states may arise in savasana, especially with continued practice – relaxation is a muscle, after all.

- Pratyahara is about turning inward. We do this by removing distractions from the space, and making ourselves as comfortable as possible so our bodies can completely relax. Then we allow all the sounds and sensations around our bodies to just be there. When our senses draw inward, our minds naturally follow – and once our mind's attention is drawn inward, there's nothing to do or fix.

- Dharana can be translated as concentration, contemplation, or reflection. When you gather your consciousness and focus on one point within yourself, there isn't room for anything else to intrude. The focus can be on an image, or your heart, or your breath, or maybe a mantra.[xii] Let this be unforced and easeful. Concentrating on softening your body with every exhale can be part of the practice of dharana.

- Dhyana is also sometimes translated as contemplation or meditation. It is when your still and quiet mind arrives at a place of unfocused and timeless awareness. An effortless state of being, not doing. Dhyana is the beginning of the union of your own dear small self with the divine and eternal, and Nischala Joy Devi calls it "the continuous inward flow of consciousness."[xiii]

- Samadhi is translated as bliss, or ecstasy, and it's a state of selfless and timeless awareness. A balanced understanding of perfect wholeness, when the illusion of separateness between the individual and the divine dissolves. One translation is "put together" – all the disparate facets unite in a state of contentment and bliss.

Sounds lovely, doesn't it? Not only are your body, mind, and spirit in harmony with each other, but you are in harmony with the greater world around you, one with all human experience and whatever higher power resonates with you. This feeling might last as long as the space between the inhale and exhale – but once it has become available, you are changed forever.

\*\*\*

If this is all too abstract, I have two more concrete images to offer you for contemplation.

The lotus is the classic image of spiritual transformation: it grows out of the mud and murk, drawing energy from within until it can burst up and open towards the light, unmuddied and clear. The blossoming lotus is a beautiful image of thriving in adverse circumstances, of expanding into glorious potential, and a great place to rest your awareness as you go deeper into meditative states.

And...

Sometimes when I am in a restorative savasana, I like to think of myself less like a lotus and more like a potato.

A potato! Nestled into the earth, growing while nobody's looking. Heavy and solid, snuggled down in the dark. A potato isn't empty calories – it can sustain a person for a long time. It's dense with potential. And adaptable! Think of all the things a potato can become!

You can be a lotus AND a potato. You can practice like the sages of thousands of years ago, another link in the same chain, stilling the mind like the Sutras guide us to do. AND you can be yourself, lying down while the world keeps spinning, gathering your resources while you let go of your burdens.

Because change is an inside job.

The more you lie down and consciously relax, the more you become attuned to how judgment physically hardens you, tightens you up, and freezes your energy. It then becomes more difficult to judge others, and to judge yourself, when you can FEEL the tension it causes in your body.

Hatred, racism, fear, creating hierarchies – it all FEELS BAD in our bodies.

Forgiveness FEELS BETTER.

*Love feels better.*

The more time we spend softening and melting the icebergs of old frozen tension in our bodies, the more we remember our true state – one with the universe and all in it.

# Coming off the mat...

## *Take your whole self with you*

After 20 minutes or longer, take your time to make your way out of the shape. If you want to do it without a timer, yoga teacher and author Judith Lasater has another option: "Practice until gratitude spontaneously arises."[xiv]

Take as long as you need to return to the rest of your life. And bring what you learned, felt, and experienced with you, because that's what we're here for.

We are here to love ourselves and each other equally and with wide open hearts, to alleviate our own suffering and the suffering of others.

We are here to wake up to the incredible joy of being alive in our own amazing bodies.

You already have everything you need to be perfect, because you are already perfect.

Please remember it!

And rest. It can change the world.

The Rest Manifesto

# Further reading

This tiny book was inspired by the work of Judith Lasater, Jillian Pransky, and my incredible teacher Adeline Tien. Please seek out their books and classes for a more comprehensive restorative experience.

Please also seek out the meditation classes provided by Michael Bruffee, Jaslyn Kee, and Suraya Sam. These wise teachers have helped me get to a place where the creation of this book was possible.

I am also influenced by Tara Brach, Sylvia Boorstein, Jack Kornfield, and Sharon Salzberg, and highly recommend their books as well – in addition to all the work mentioned in the endnotes.

And if you are on the path of Reiki, please check out the books of my teacher Elaine Hamilton Grundy.

# Gratitude

I am eternally grateful to so many people for being part of my sangha. Adeline Tien, for introducing me to restorative yoga. Sophie Sanders, for her sunny guidance and wise encouragement. Dr. Anne Wenstrom for the opportunity to teach, and Ana María Gach for being an early and supportive student. I am also so grateful for the guidance and community of Dr. Trish Rice Corley and the Thunderbolts.

Thanks to all my writing groups: the Freeskate crew from Emerson (Ben Gould, Nayiri Krikorian, Marcella Hammer, Audubon Dougherty, Greg Campbell, Jen Heller); One Two Three Floor from Singapore (Rebecca Clark, Jen Megee, Scott Riley, Matt Elms), and the Bitches Who Write. I couldn't have done this without their encouragement, and without the loving container created by the Tiny Book crew.

Extra double thanks to Nayiri Krikorian for her gimlet eye, and to an economic botany exhibit I once saw in DC about potatoes.

Above all, thanks to my parents, my brother, and my whole family for their unwavering support and belief, and Bob Helmer for being the greatest human being of all time. You inspire me every day, BH.

# About the author

Beth Bayley is a certified vinyasa and restorative yoga teacher, poet, baker, and occasional archivist, just trying to do her best to get everyone to lie down. Her work has been published in Slant, vox poetica, Green Hills Literary Lantern, and the Evening Street Review, among others. She lives in Singapore and Massachusetts with her husband. Find more at bethbayley.yoga.

# Endnotes

---

[i] My parents claim to not remember this, but I do!

[ii] Or maybe it was 2001 (the mists of time, etc.), at the long gone Baptiste Power Yoga Studio in on Columbus Ave in Boston, and the teacher was the marvelous Rolf Gates.

[iii] Stephen Cope's *The Great Work of Your Life: A Guide for the Journey to Your True Calling* (Bantam, 2015) is a good read on this topic.

[iv] Not that there's anywhere to get. Or that we really know where we're going.

[v] Dr. Herbert Benson introduced the concept of the Relaxation Response in his 1975 book of the same name. The response naturally arises after 20 minutes of feeling safe, and breathing in a relaxed manner with no muscular effort or tension.

[vi] You can do them later! You are here now.

[vii] Via the research of Dr. Jill Bolte Taylor, author of *My Stroke of Insight: A Brain Scientist's Personal Journey* (Penguin, 2009).

[viii] For more on this, see *Your Body Speaks Your Mind* by Deb Shapiro (Sounds True, 2006), as well as the work of Reiki Master teacher Elaine Hamilton Grundy.

[ix] From Tara Brach's *Radical Acceptance: Embracing Your Life with the Heart of a Buddha* (Bantam, 2003), p. 42

[x] Though I don't know that the way is necessarily linear. Human beings are more inclined toward circles and meandering than we are to straight lines.

[xi] A description of all the Sutras is outside the scope of this small book, but please do read them and read up on them – new and excellent resources are coming out all the time.

[xii] This can be very simple – a mantra can just be a word that you like, one that evokes positive feelings in your body. Repeat it to yourself as you exhale, allowing yourself and the word to become one.

[xiii] *The Secret Power of Yoga: A Woman's Guide to the Heart and Spirit of the Yoga Sutras* by Nischala Joy Devi, (Three Rivers, 2007), p. 251

[xiv] Via *Conversations with a Yogi* podcast, Jan 21 2019.